# THE WHOLESOME DIET

## By:NEIL W BARLOW

ISBN: 978-1-300-96267-0

www.publishnation.co.uk

# INTRODUCTION

'Diet' as defined in the Shorter Oxford English Dictionary means a) a way of <u>living</u> or <u>thinking</u> and b) a way of <u>feeding</u>. I hope to address all sides of this subject as briefly and succinctly as possible.

It isn't that easy to diet: if it were, everyone would do it and no one would have any further concerns.

Moreover it is only ever a part of your whole life to start and keep up a diet.

Every one of you is different, with your own reasons for even considering a diet. Men and women have very different approaches, the former going for all-or-nothing and the latter adopting a gradual process.

There is however one constant theme – the search for a weight and shape which suits your lifestyle and body image. If you are honest with yourself, it is also about looking as beautiful as possible.

The human form varies enormously, and scientific measurements such as Body-Mass-Index (BMI) are of limited value. There is however one test we can all do. Pick up 1Kg of sugar and carry it upstairs. Do you really not care about all your extra weight?

Much is made of the role of exercise in helping to achieve a better weight and shape. I will argue that exercise is the catalyst to self-improvement, making you look and feel better, and jump-starting the dieting process. It will not however work on its own. The same is true of dieting.

The first step is for you to choose a target weight for yourself. You should be realistic about this, neither making it too demanding nor too easy to achieve. It is important that it is a possible target, taking into account your lifestyle, work, health, family and other pressures. If the target is expressed as a round number in kilograms, pounds or stones, it will be easy to remember.

This book on diet will not cost you much money and may in fact save you unnecessary expenditure. Results will be seen quickly and targets achieved within a year. There is no knowing what you can do with a little help, and I am sure that you will realise your ambitions for yourself.

# YOUR PERSONAL PHILOSOPHY

We all have a personal philosophy of life. It is just that, like God and religion, we don't care to think about it too often. It comes to the fore at certain times in our lives, such as leaving home, middle age and retirement. In fact, like money, it needs more frequent attention than we give it.

So let's consider what needs to be in your personal philosophy. Your physical health and appearance inevitably come first because of being always on show, to yourself and to others.

Are you blessed with good health or have you had to make adjustments to cope with failings? Are you good-looking, average, or do you have some bad features? What stature and shape are you? Whatever the answer to these questions, be assured that no one is ever happy with the way they look, but it is important to make the best of what you look like. Why not take the obvious steps towards improving or maintaining your health and shape, rather than wait for someone else to tell you? One action taken of your own volition is worth many times the actions you take on the advice of experts in the medical or other professions.

What no one will tell you, and also you cannot usually work out for yourself, are your good

3

features. You will always have some of these which others envy, and which are peculiar to yourself. You yourself do not rate them, because you have always had them and assume that others do too. Try to appreciate them if you can.

You have an image of yourself when you buy clothes, which may range from extreme pessimism to heady optimism. To start your diet you will have to work out what is possible and practicable.

The amount of exercise you take is influenced by so many factors, such as your genes, upbringing, time of life and competing interests and opportunities. I warn you however that exercise is necessary!

So let us assume that you have developed a reasonable working self-image of yourself, involving an attainable weight, appearance, shape and physical presence, and can imagine a healthy lifestyle involving exercise. What else is necessary to complete your personal philosophy?

Without an appropriate mental approach no diet will be successful. A healthy mind in a healthy body ('mens sana in corpore sano' as the Romans had it) is a good recipe for success. Why you originally wanted to diet may not matter: but to continue and achieve a result needs a mental discipline able to deliver the required 'mind over matter'. So many external influences preach the opposite, glorifying the body and advocating a hedonistic lifestyle. Self-indulgence may even be a work requirement in some jobs. However if you want to be your own person, it will not be difficult for you to contradict these influences.

Some people find that an external body – a church, society, club or association – is helpful to them in setting out clear rules and providing a disciplined environment. Some rely on family or friends to provide the honest feedback they need. However there are two essential steps you must take before you can reduce food intake and increase exercise. You have to a) admit you are overweight and b) will yourself to take the necessary steps to remedy your condition.

The personal philosophy goes yet further than physical self-image and discipline of mind. You must also have a belief in your ability to succeed. This is really a gift – whether by grace from above, or from your nature or from your upbringing. If you are willing to be receptive, you will be guided by a kind of sixth sense away from being overweight and towards a proper size and shape. Depending on your character, you may adopt a Platonist or an Aristotelian route to your target. The former postulates an absolute standard of truth and beauty, to which to aspire. The latter prefers a golden mean of virtue which is gradually achieved by small steps, sometimes forward and sometimes backward when things go wrong. Either approach will work for you in developing self-belief.

The personal philosophy is therefore composed of three things – self-image, self-discipline and self-belief.

# PHYSICAL ASPECTS: (a) Diet

So it is Day 1 of your new life and you are considering the vast range of diets on offer. Before spending a lot of money or entering into long-term contracts, consider just how much external stimulus and support you really need. Many of us are not motivated by a bunch of other fallible human beings and prefer to go it alone. The good news is that this route is free of charge and brings its own reward for achieving a tough challenge on your own. Social scientists have demonstrated how people seek to satisfy their basic needs first – for food, shelter and security – but then strive for self-development and self-actualisation, to be the best that you can be. If these last two are attained autonomously, on your own, they are more likely to last.

Many more of us however need a guide and a support group to get started. Spending money on a programme may represent the first concrete commitment made towards starting a diet. There is no harm in this, but it is not a very powerful catalyst compared with a purely personal commitment to diet. Such groups and their leaders do wield a number of quite effective carrots and sticks. These range from the award of gold stars, price discounts, titles and applause, to the sanction of public naming and shaming when extra pounds have been gained. Many people start and stop their diets with bewildering regularity and rapidity, believing that dieting is simply a matter of eating less or differently. They believe there is a magic fix for their overweight.

A great deal of money has been made by the proponents of these diets. One of these had many adherents despite its reputation for causing halitosis – until the founder died in middle age. It is less popular now.

The truth is that the body is a machine which needs a certain amount of fuel. If it is filled up too full or too often, it cannot burn off the surplus on ordinary activities and hence will add to your girth and your weight. Most people eat too much, especially older people, and would benefit from occasional fasting. The presence of sugar and other additives in our food and drink makes it all that much harder. Eating and drinking the right amount is very difficult in our busy and sociable lives. Fortunately lapses do not matter and treats are to be encouraged, provided that the overall objective of a sensible weight and shape is not damaged.

Just starting a diet and hoping for a miracle is a common practice. More sophisticated dieters may establish detailed targets and obtain feedback on their progress. Some will even weigh every particle of food and drink and assess its calorific value, before it passes their lips. As with any enterprise, involving a journey from A to B, it is essential to set some milestones on the way as well as the ultimate target. Some broad-brush measures will suffice in my view, particularly as the body will experience natural fluctuations due to health, wellbeing, social and family pressures, and the stresses and strains of ordinary working life. Do not worry about minor deviations as long as the general trend is favourable.

Let us assume that your diet works perfectly for you. You are eating and drinking more healthily, more moderately and more consistently, but you are still not losing very much weight. What else is needed?

# PHYSICAL ASPECTS:
# (b) Exercise

The answer is physical exertion, which together with food and drink forms the tripartite balance necessary to achieve a good weight and shape. Young children find that lots of activity and good basic food and drink give a natural balance without any need for attention. Anorexia, bulimia and obesity are caused by other factors in an otherwise healthy child. Self-image problems generally start only in the teens and will decrease in intensity with maturity. Role models, both the accepted and rejected ones, are important at this stage and should be carefully monitored by the parents, as part of their overall duty of care.

Adults are different, with money, time and freedom to do what they like. Some binge on food and drink and take no exercise. Some subject their bodies to all kinds of hardship including extreme exercise. Social life and work bring a lack of care for our bodies. Then, usually in young middle-age, comes the realisation that youth and health are no longer a 'given'. They are not eternal and nor are we. Decisions about lifestyle come to the fore. Those who are married with children often settle into a comfortable and expected acceptance of their overweight, seeing it as part of a parent or grandparent's image in society. It is left to the unmarried to worry about their health and appearance. In today's world, when one in three marriages break down, such thinking is old-fashioned; and in any case can it ever have been right? To be of reasonably attractive appearance is possible throughout your life, even if it does require more attention as you grow older. Exercise is a matter of personal taste, means and availability. Some like extreme sports such as fell-running, hang-gliding or deep-sea diving. Others like walking, cycling and swimming which are normally within everyone's reach. Being a couch potato is not exercise or sport at any age!

However you choose to exercise your body, why not make it as congenial and enjoyable as possible? In the gym you can meet others, set competitive targets, or listen to your favourite music while developing the body beautiful. In the open air, you can take an interest in the surrounding landscape with its flora and fauna, sun, rain, wind and clouds, on top of the benefits you obtain indoors. Only prolonged and vigorous exercise will have a noticeable effect on your weight by itself.

Exercise also has another important function. To start off on your self-improvement, a catalyst is required. Do something exceptional with your body, like a charity swim, a cycle or a moonlight walk. The resulting euphoria will well outlive the aches and pains, and prove to you in a singular and dramatic way that you can achieve improvement, that through a gradual process you will be able to build on it, and that you have already started your exercise regime.

# PHYSICAL ASPECTS:
# (c) Diet and Exercise

The secret to achieving and maintaining your ideal weight and shape and health depends on the correct balance for you of diet and exercise. You find this out by experience, by trial and error and by simply living your normal life. You can eat steak pies, pizzas and fried potatoes if you are climbing several hills at the weekend, training for highly competitive sports such as rowing, or indeed if it is a special one–off treat for your birthday.

If however your exercise is a gentle walk, yoga or sailing a comfortable yacht or cruiser, then eating fatty things will soon push up your weight. It is a question of balance.

The measurement fiends will have their calories monitored both for diet and exercise. This is wholly understandable and wholly unnecessary. A rough rule of thumb is all that is needed. Furthermore there may be certain foods such as chocolate, and certain drinks such as wine, which in practice may hardly make any difference to weight in your case.

Everyone is different and has a unique key to diet and exercise.

# MENTAL ASPECTS

Mind over matter is not easy to achieve but it is an essential part of dieting. Our bodies tell us to eat when we are hungry or drink when thirsty. The rest of it is down to habit, with gluttony and sloth calling the shots – unless we control the habit and bring abstinence and energy to our aid.

Habits are useful in everyday living, and you may feel daunted about the challenge of changing them; but they are easy to change with willpower. Try it yourself – instead of two lumps of sugar in your tea or coffee, take one or none for a week. The heavens will not fall in and you may even feel better. Addiction is a different matter, but fortunately tea, coffee and even alcohol are not seriously addictive for most people. The cause of much self-indulgence is boredom, and this can be fixed. Holidays and suchlike rarely change habits, because you are carrying round with you the same mental attitude. Applying your brain direct to your problem is the only way to solve it.

So take a hard look at your eating, drinking and exercising habits. At the same time take a look at the rest of your habits – TV, sleep, sex, work and recreation. All would benefit from a break in the habits built up over many years, usually for sound reasons. Questioning your previously successful strategies is the hardest thing to do. If it works, don't change it! However the point is that it is not working to your satisfaction, in that you cannot achieve the weight and shape you want.

The mind and body are closely connected but operate separately and in their own ways. The body feels pain or pleasure directly, but the mind is more complex. It has its own thoughts and expectations, and the mismatch between these and what is actually happening is called feelings. For example, happiness is unexpected pleasure while anger and frustration arise from the mismatch of expectation and reality. Thus body and mind are perpetually adjusting to each other as a result of their own experiences. It is not abnormal for one to dictate to the other and for the other to respond.

Is it desirable to have a body and mind in perpetual harmony? Contented cows are not necessarily productive or achieving their best output. In humans a 'divine discontent' will always operate to prevent low goals from being set and achieved with ease. Striving for perfection and being dissatisfied with less is hardwired into us. Therefore the mind will always be aware of the shortcomings of the body, and within reason this is normal and manageable. It is however easy to go overboard on criticism of your own body, setting impossible targets or despairing of any improvement. A steady and sustainable improvement is possible if you give your mind to it.

So how do you go about applying your brain to changing your bad habits and encouraging your good ones? Analysis of how you spend your time and money is a good place to start. Do you get up late, loll around all day and then try to do everything in the evening? Is your eating and drinking excessive, highly irregular or inadequate and inessential nourishment?

Do you have to have a certain type of mind or intelligence to control your body? Does it require special training? Is it really difficult?

The answer is no to all three questions. It is easy to exaggerate the scale of your own problem, underestimate your own good qualities, and doubt the strength of your commitment. You have realised that you are carrying too much weight and decided to do something about it. Both body and brain are capable of so much more than we demand of them. See how things get done if you have limited time, if your objective is clear and if there is sufficient incentive. A war scenario gives a perfect example.

Commitment to a course of action involves choice: by choosing to do A, you rule out or postpone B, C and D. Thus time or lack of it is never an excuse for inaction: you just do not want the result enough to give it priority over your other activities. Once you have decided on a diet and started the process, can anything stop you? Unfortunately it can.

In business terms there are very low hurdles to entry on a dieting programme. This means that it is easy to start, but not that it is easy to keep up. Your body starts objecting to the lack of its normal food and drink. It may register hollowness, even hunger. Your mind is meanwhile in a quandary. It remembers its commitment to dieting but it does not like the feelings arising from the body's dissatisfaction with the policy. It casts about for alternative strategies, rationalisations for why it should pander to the body just this once and questions how important it all is. It wants to get its peace of mind at any cost. This discomfort is far, far worse than the bodily result of eating less. It has to be overcome and does test the commitment you have. Each challenge by the body will have the same effect on the mind. Each assault has to be fought off, occasionally unsuccessfully but with increasing confidence. No surrender is final, you always live to fight another day. You can lose a battle and still win the war.

Compared with the body, which has certain needs and capacities which are reasonably straightforward and understandable, the mind is full of tricks. Nothing is ever finally decided or resolved; it is always subject to new evidence or influence, not necessarily for good. So your commitment to the diet will come under intellectual as well as physical assault. There is a new improved diet which should be tried but which means abandoning your existing diet, often with disastrous consequences. You give up the gym to try out a more sophisticated exercise schedule. You meet someone new who undermines your belief in your previous actions. No one is immune to these intellectual challenges but none of it changes the basic proposition which brought you to your diet in the first place.

Then there are the heavy guns which at the very least will bring about a pause or postponement of your project. Accident, emergency, serious illness, bankruptcy, family troubles – all these and more are genuinely a reason to abandon your diet. Let us hope they do not happen. The truth is often more mundane and your diet is given up for inadequate and insubstantial reasons. The body and mind capitulate to a paper tiger.

You need reinforcement – and this is called the spiritual dimension. With it you can and will succeed.

# SPIRITUAL ASPECTS

There seems to be little connection between your religious beliefs and your diet. God does not care about your weight and shape. The spiritual life is a completely separate matter.

None of these statements is true. How your body feels, what meals you eat, and your exercise choices are all important components of your religious beliefs, however feeble these may be. Orders of monks and nuns prescribe both eating and activity, and many religions such as Judaism have many rules affecting these areas of life. Even if you do not subscribe to organised religion and do not believe in God, you will have some basic spiritual tenets which govern your life. If you have no such tenets and live a life of pure anarchy, you are quite a rarity. Many behave in an immoral or amoral way, but are still aware of the morals they fail to live by.
The Greeks and Romans provide perhaps the best documented examples of how to combine all aspects of body, mind and spirit together in pursuit of a good life. Typical of Greek culture was the attempt to set boundaries on our bodily appetites as part of the good life. We can perhaps label this as a pagan or pre-Christian beliefs. Such values and many others form the ramshackle set of principles many of us live by.

We are not often aware of these principles except in periods of physical or mental stress such as serious ill-health. There are also certain times in our lives when we contemplate our mortality and measure ourselves and our achievements. This may take the form of a list of targets which derive from the expectations of our parents, ourselves or of others. There will be measures of health and happiness, financial success and development of our talents both in work and leisure.

The assessment can start with your weight and shape but you will soon find it necessary to include other less tangible factors such as health and happiness. In defining them you realise how you are made up of complex and diverse influences, which form your personality. They all inter-relate and they all affect your ability to find and stick to a diet and exercise regime.

These are difficult topics for most of us, and yet you will have to tackle them sooner or later. Women usually want to look beautiful and attractive, and this provides the key incentive to diet. Men know that they are less likely to look either of the above, or else they rank beauty below other traits like manliness, risk-taking and sporting success.

Determining your spiritual toolkit in this way is a big step on the road to a successful diet. Conversely if your fundamental beliefs are at odds with your decision to diet and exercise, you will have no chance of success. To take an extreme example, a fatalistic approach to life (nothing I do matters since it is all predetermined) will give you no encouragement whatsoever.

If however you believe that you are responsible for yourself, that it is important to make the best of your life here and now, and that your body is important since you are a part of nature and respond to natural impulses, then it is incumbent on you to look after your body.

# MEASURING SUCCESS

I have left this until last, but actually it is essential at every stage of the diet to get feedback in an appropriate form, so that you can act on it by modifying your behaviour.

The first obvious measures are the mirror and the weighing machine. Both should be consulted daily at a fixed time. Most convenient times are bed-times and getting-up times, but it is for you to choose. Clearly you have to be wearing the same clothing in order to achieve consistency of results. It does not matter whether you use kilograms, stones or pounds, provided that you bear in mind your target look and your target weight. These should be written down somewhere for reference. The result of your daily weigh-in should be recorded in a diary, and soon you will come to realise which foods are to be avoided (except as a treat) and which exercise is most effective in delivering your desired shape and size.

Everyone is different, and the optimal mix of diet and exercise for you is only achieved by trial and error. Your weight will drop if you undertake strenuous exercise, but it will be balanced out by the food you eat. Weight is never stable. It is either on a rising or a falling trend, and hunts up and down like automatic heating controls, often for quite inexplicable reasons linked to your metabolism, health, anxiety or stress. Over the years however, once you have achieved target weight, you will understand the pattern to some extent.

This feedback loop will contribute to your morale either positively or negatively, but it cannot be ignored. It will help you to develop a well-judged diet and healthy eating habits.

Be advised against highly sophisticated measures. There is so much we do not understand about our bodies that a too detailed reading will frequently dismay or confuse you. Just choose a regular routine method and stick to it through thick and thin.

# ENDPIECE

I hope you have enjoyed this highly individual approach to dieting. It focuses on a holistic theme involving body, mind and spirit. It can be highly effective.

Your desired weight, shape and image may seem trivial to you, but after all we live with ourselves all the year round, every waking minute, and observe our own flaws every day. Frequently we underestimate our own advantages. My aim has been to give you a fighting chance of success, whatever your age and circumstances, of achieving the body of your dreams and keeping it so, all your life long.

# Performance Record

# Performance Record

# Performance Record

# Performance Record

# Performance Record

# Performance Record

# Performance Record